# Pediatric Test of Brain Injury™ (PTBI™) TEST FORM

Gillian Hotz, Nancy Helm-Estabrooks,
Nickola Wolf Nelson, and Elena Plante

PTBI

## CHILD'S INFORMATION

Child's name: ______________________

Case/medical record ID number: ______________________

Child's city and state: ______________________

Child's school: ______________________

Child's grade: ______________________

Child's gender: ___ female ___ male

Language(s) spoken: ___ English ___ Spanish

___ Other: ______________________

Classroom performance (prior to injury):

___ below average ___ average ___ above average

Handedness: ___ right ___ left ___ ambidextrous

Any hand restrictions due to injury: ______________________

Any speaking restrictions due to injury (e.g., intubation):__________

______________________

| | Year | Month | Day | | Year | Month | Day |
|---|---|---|---|---|---|---|---|
| Date tested | | | | Date tested | | | |
| Date of birth | | | | Date of injury/onset | | | |
| Chronological age | | | | Time post-injury/onset | | | |

*Note:* Subtract date of birth from date tested to get chronological age. Subtract date of injury/onset from date tested to get time post-injury/onset.

## TESTING INFORMATION

Examiner's name: ______________________

Facility: ______________________

## MEDICAL HISTORY

AF753067

Primary diagnosis: __________

Mechanism of injury: __________

GCS[1] on admission: __________

GCS[1] at PTBI testing: ______________________

RLAS[2] at PTBI testing: ______________________

CT/MRI results: ______________________

______________________

Surgical procedures: ______________________

______________________

Current medications: ______________________

______________________

______________________

Previous head injury: ___ yes ___ no

Other prior problems (specify): ______________________

[1]*Glasgow Coma Scale* [2]*Rancho Los Amigos Scale*

***NOTE:*** *If the PTBI is administered in two sessions, they must be* ***on the same day.*** *The first session must end after Subtest 5; the second session begins with Subtest 6.*

Testing time: Session 1 _______ Session 2 _______

Total testing time: ___________

| SUMMARY SCORING CHART | Ability Score (from Test Form) | Performance Category (from Appendix A) | *SEM* | Confidence Interval | Previous Test Results | |
|---|---|---|---|---|---|---|
| **Constrained Skills** | | **VL** = Very Low **L** = Low **M** = Moderate **H** = High | Standard error of measurement (from Appendix B) | Add and subtract *SEM* from Ability Score | Date: ________ Ability Score | Perf. Category |
| 1. Orientation | _____ | ❒ VL ❒ L ❒ M ❒ H | _____ | _____ to _____ | _____ | _____ |
| 2. Following Commands | _____ | ❒ VL ❒ L ❒ M ❒ H | _____ | _____ to _____ | _____ | _____ |
| 6. Naming | _____ | ❒ VL ❒ L ❒ M ❒ H | _____ | _____ to _____ | _____ | _____ |
| **Unconstrained Skills** | | | | | | |
| 3. Word Fluency | _____ | ❒ VL ❒ L ❒ M ❒ H | _____ | _____ to _____ | _____ | _____ |
| 4. What Goes Together | _____ | ❒ VL ❒ L ❒ M ❒ H | _____ | _____ to _____ | _____ | _____ |
| 5. Digit Span | _____ | ❒ VL ❒ L ❒ M ❒ H | _____ | _____ to _____ | _____ | _____ |
| 7. Story Retelling—Immediate | _____ | ❒ VL ❒ L ❒ M ❒ H | _____ | _____ to _____ | _____ | _____ |
| 8. Yes/No/Maybe | _____ | ❒ VL ❒ L ❒ M ❒ H | _____ | _____ to _____ | _____ | _____ |
| 9. Picture Recall | _____ | ❒ VL ❒ L ❒ M ❒ H | _____ | _____ to _____ | _____ | _____ |
| 10. Story Retelling—Delayed | _____ | ❒ VL ❒ L ❒ M ❒ H | _____ | _____ to _____ | _____ | _____ |

**SUMMARY OF OVERALL PERFORMANCE:** ______________________________________

## ATTENTION EXAMINERS

**Before administering this test:**

- Read Chapter 5 in the *PTBI Examiner's Manual.*
- Study the testing procedures so that you can administer the PTBI accurately and smoothly.
- Do not test individuals who are agitated or upset.
- Under no circumstances should you use PTBI tasks for practice or treatment.

**For valid, standardized testing:**

- *Do not vary* from PTBI administration procedures as they are written in the PTBI Test Form.
- Administer all PTBI subtests in the order they appear.
- Discontinue testing if individuals become agitated or upset during testing.
- Do not discuss PTBI performance with examinees during administration. If examinees ask how they are doing, say, "We can talk about that after we're finished."
- Do not tell examinees whether their responses were correct or incorrect.
- Do not provide leading questions, prompts, or probes that may serve as cues.
- Use only those questions, prompts, and probes as stated in the instruction banner of each subtest.
- If giving the test in two sessions, end Session 1 at Subtest 5 (Digit Span) and begin Session 2 with Subtest 6 (Naming).
- Always conduct the two sessions on the same day.
- Do not deviate from specific directions for subtest administration and for recording and scoring responses as printed in the instruction banners.

**Prompts and probes:**

- A *prompt* is a neutral form of encouragement (e.g., "You can keep going," "We have to move along," "You have time to check your work"). During testing, use only neutral prompts such as "We're moving along" or "Only a few more."
- A *probe* is a cue for more specific information (e.g., "What is your *last* name?").
- Use only those prompts and probes that appear in instruction banners.

## SUBTEST 1: ORIENTATION

**Materials** Test Form

**Instructions** Say, ***"First, I need to find out some things about you."*** Record the child's responses verbatim.

*Probe:* For last name and month, day, and year, as necessary

*Note:* If the child cannot speak, accept written responses on a separate sheet. Attach written responses to Test Form.

**Discontinue Rule** None

**Repetition** If the child asks or does not respond within 10 seconds, each item may be repeated once.

**Scoring**
- Cross out ability score for any incorrect item; circle ability score for each correct item.
- Add scores for correct items to compute total ability score.

| Item | Question/Response | Ability Score |
|---|---|---|
| 1 | ***What is your full name?*** (Child must say both first and last name. If child does not say last name on first trial, **probe** for last name.) | 0.5 |
| 2 | ***How old are you?*** | 1.5 |
| 3a | ***When is your birthday?*** (For incomplete responses, **probe** for month, day, and year.) Month | 2.0 |
| 3b | Day | 2.0 |
| 3c | Year | 3.5 |
| 4 | ***What grade are you in?*** (If summer, accept either completed or upcoming grade.) | 2.0 |
| 5 | ***What school do you go to?*** | 3.0 |
| 6 | ***What city or town do you live in?*** (If rural address, accept nearest town.) | 4.0 |
| 7 | ***What state/province do you live in?*** | 3.5 |
| 8 | ***What is this place?*** (Accept "hospital," "clinic," "school," "home," and so forth.) | 3.5 |
| 9 | ***What day of the week is it today?*** | 4.5 |
| 10 | ***What month is it?*** | 4.0 |
| 11 | ***What year is it?*** | 4.0 |

Time to administer: _____ **TOTAL ORIENTATION ABILITY SCORE** _____ / 38.0

**Behavioral observations:** (Abbreviations may be used next to items where they apply.)

___ Repetition of instructions (Rep)
___ Attention reminder required (Attn)
___ Prompt to reestablish set (Prompt)
___ Perseveration (P)
___ Delayed response (5+ sec) (DR)
___ Unintelligible response (UnR)
___ No response (NR)
___ I don't know (IDK)
___ Self-correction (SC)

**Additional qualitative/behavioral observations:**

**Notes for examiners on Orientation:** Orientation to person, place, and date is a key component of any examination of individuals with brain injury. By recording exact responses, you can look for behaviors, such as perseveration of earlier responses and patterns such as disorientation to time but not person or place. Individuals may have response difficulties secondary to word retrieval and production.

## SUBTEST 2: FOLLOWING COMMANDS

**Materials** Test Form

**Instructions** Say, ***"Okay, now I want you to do some things without talking. Wait until I finish telling you what to do before you start. Here's one for practice."***

*Practice item:* ***"Close your eyes."*** (If the child's eyes stay shut, say, ***"Okay, now open them."***)

Record deviations from each required (underlined) component. The child must demonstrate all required components in the sequence specified to receive credit.

**Discontinue Rule** None

**Repetition** If the child asks or does not respond within 10 seconds, each command may be repeated once.

**Scoring**
- Cross out ability score for any item not completely correct; circle ability score for each correct item.
- Add scores for correct items to compute total ability score.

| Item | Command/Response | Ability Score |
|---|---|---|
| 1 | ***Where's your knee?*** | 0.5 |
| 2 | ***Make a fist.*** | 1.5 |
| 3 | ***Stick out your tongue and then point to the door.*** | 1.5 |
| 4 | ***Before you point to the floor, point to your foot.*** | 1.5 |
| 5 | ***After you look at the ceiling, touch your heart.*** | 1.5 |
| 6 | ***With your thumb, touch your stomach.*** | 2.5 |
| 7 | ***Look to the left and then to the right.*** | 3.0 |
| 8 | ***Point to the light after you shake your head.*** | 3.0 |

Time to administer: _____ **TOTAL FOLLOWING COMMANDS ABILITY SCORE** _____ / 15.0

**Behavioral observations:** (Abbreviations may be used next to items where they apply.)

| | | |
|---|---|---|
| ___ Repetition of instructions (Rep) | ___ Perseveration (P) | ___ No response (NR) |
| ___ Attention reminder required (Attn) | ___ Delayed response (5+ sec) (DR) | ___ I don't know (IDK) |
| ___ Prompt to reestablish set (Prompt) | ___ Unintelligible response (UnR) | ___ Self-correction (SC) |

**Additional qualitative/behavioral observations:**

**Notes for examiners on Following Commands:** The ability to accurately follow commands is crucial for both rehabilitation and educational programs. Although examiners often assume that level of difficulty can be accounted for simply by length, item response theory analysis for this test indicated otherwise (as reflected in the scoring system). Record examinees' exact responses so that you can look for behavioral patterns such as perseveration (e.g., pointing again to a particular object) and sequencing problems.

## SUBTEST 3: WORD FLUENCY

### 3A. Semantic: Animals

**Materials** Test Form, Stimulus Book (page 1), watch with second hand or stopwatch

**Instructions** **This subtest is timed.** 60 seconds is allowed for each part.

Show the printed word ***ANIMALS*** to the child. Leave the stimulus page open for the duration of the task.

Say, ***"I want you to name as many animals as you can in 1 minute. Can you think of an animal?"***

- If the child names an animal, say, ***"Good. Name as many animals as you can. Start now."*** (Start timing and write words the child says in the box for the appropriate time interval.)
- If the child stops before the minute is up, prompt, ***"Keep going. You have more time."***
- Only prompt once, but keep timing until the 60 seconds is up.

**Discontinue Rule** None

**Repetition** If the child asks or does not respond within 10 seconds, repeat the directions once.

**Scoring**

- Count each correct new animal named.
- Any animal or category counts (e.g., mammals, insects, birds, dinosaurs).
- Count semantic variants (e.g., *sow* and *pig* count as 2; *African elephant* and *Indian elephant* count as 2; but *baby elephant* and *big elephant* count as 1).
- Diminutive or plural forms of the same word count as 1 (e.g., *dog* and *doggie*; *cat* and *cats*).
- Do not count any word that is not an animal, is perseverated (mark P), or is a nonword.
- Do not penalize dysarthria (e.g., *agillator*) or recognizable mispronunciations (e.g., *elevant*).
- Score 1 point for each acceptable response.

| 0–15 seconds | 16–30 seconds | 31–45 seconds | 46–60 seconds |
|---|---|---|---|
| | | | |

**Animal Fluency Score** _____

### 3B. Phonemic: *M* words

**Materials** Test Form, Stimulus Book (page 2)

**Instructions** Show the printed letter ***M*** to the child and leave the stimulus page open for the duration of the task.

Say, ***"I want you to name as many words beginning with the letter* M *as you can in 1 minute. The letter* M *says /mmmm/. Can you think of a word starting with the letter* M?"**

- If the child names a word beginning with *M,* say, ***"Good. Name as many* M *words as you can. Start now."*** (Start timing and write words the child says in the box for the appropriate time interval.)
- If the child stops before the minute is up, prompt him or her by saying, ***"Keep going. You have more time."***
- Only prompt once, but keep timing until the 60 seconds is up.

**Discontinue Rule** None

**Repetition** If the child asks or does not respond within 10 seconds, repeat the directions once.

**Scoring**

- Count each correct new *M* word produced.
- Count proper names.
- Count each derivative form (e.g., *mom, mommy,* and *mother* count as 3) but not inflected forms such as plurals (*mom* and *moms* count as 1) or inflected verb forms (*make* and *making* count as 1).
- Do not count any word that is not an *M* word, is perseverated (mark P), or is a nonword.
- Do not penalize dysarthria or recognizable mispronunciations.
- Score 1 point for each acceptable response.
- Compute total ability score by adding scores for both parts of the subtest.

| 0–15 seconds | 16–30 seconds | 31–45 seconds | 46–60 seconds |
|---|---|---|---|
| | | | |

*M* **Fluency Score** ____

**Animal Fluency Score** ____

**TOTAL WORD FLUENCY SCORE** ____

**Behavioral observations:** (Abbreviations may be used next to items where they apply.)

| | | |
|---|---|---|
| ___ Repetition of instructions (Rep) | ___ Perseveration (P) | ___ No response (NR) |
| ___ Attention reminder required (Attn) | ___ Delayed response (5+ sec) (DR) | ___ I don't know (IDK) |
| ___ Prompt to reestablish set (Prompt) | ___ Unintelligible response (UnR) | ___ Self-correction (SC) |

**Additional qualitative/behavioral observations:**

**Notes for examiners on Word Fluency:** Word Fluency calls on multiple cognitive-linguistic skills involved in conducting an organized mental search by category, so this task is a sensitive measure of brain function. Review recorded responses for qualitative observations of performance. Positive executive behaviors include the use of subcategories of animals to aid word retrieval. Look also for negative behaviors, such as perseveration (repetition of an earlier response), as this behavior is associated with brain dysfunction. By entering responses according to time intervals, you can see whether there is consistent recall across the intervals, a warm-up effect, or quick exhaustion of the mental search. Other negative behaviors include "loss-of-set" (failure to stay on task) and partial "stuck-in-set" (e.g., naming only animals that begin with the letter *M*).

## SUBTEST 4: WHAT GOES TOGETHER

**Materials** Test Form, Stimulus Book (pages 3–10)

**Instructions** *Practice item:* Begin by training the child to do this task. Open the Stimulus Book to page 3 and say, ***"Here are three words. Let's read them together."*** (Reading in unison is allowed but not required.) ***"dog–cat–bone"***

Say, **"Tell me two words that go together."**

- Circle the child's responses in the lines provided.
- The order of the child's responses does not matter.

Then ask, ***"Why?"***

*Probing for the practice item:* If the response to the question ***"Why?"*** on the practice item is not a good/primary/dominant response, say, ***"Can you think of a better reason to put dog and cat*** [or dog and bone] ***together?"*** If the child does not say, "Both are animals," or another appropriate answer, probe, ***"Do you think that they are both animals? How about that for a reason?"***

*Test items:* Proceed to the test items.

Say, ***"Now you will put other words together."*** Read the words aloud. Then say, ***"What two are you putting together?"*** Then ask, ***"Why?"*** Record responses verbatim.

Then say, ***"What other two are you putting together?"*** and ***"Why?"***

Do not probe for more elaborate answers within the test items. Just ask for pairings and rationales.

*Note:* If the child is not able to speak but can write, permit written responses.

**Discontinue Rule** Discontinue testing only if the child does not respond to the practice item (all parts) or gets no credit for parts a, b, c, and d for 3 consecutive items. Cross out scores for all remaining items.

**Repetition** None

**Scoring**

- Circle the responses the child gives.
- Circle the child's reason or write in a reason that is not listed.
- Both word pairs must be correct to receive word-pair credit in column on right.
- Reasons *why* are scored separately.
- Do not credit reason for any incorrect word pair.
- Cross out ability score for any incorrect item and any items past point of discontinuation; circle ability score for each correct item.
- Add subtotals for each column.
- Compute total ability score by adding the column subscores.

**Practice**

a **dog** — **cat** — bone

b ***Why?***

both animals, both pets (**not**—dogs chase cats [not core meaning])

c **dog** — cat — **bone**

d ***Why?***

dogs like / eat / bury / chew bones

| Item | Item Content/Responses | Ability Score | Item | Item Content/Responses | Ability Score |
|---|---|---|---|---|---|
| 1a | **red** — apple — **blue** | | 1c | **red** — **apple** — blue | 0.5 |
| 1b | ***Why?*** both colors | 6.0 | 1d | ***Why?*** apple is / can be red | 6.0 |
| 2a | **knife** — **fork** — saw | | 2c | **knife** — fork — **saw** | 5.0 |
| 2b | ***Why?*** things you eat with, utensils, silverware | 2.5 | 2d | ***Why?*** both sharp, used to cut | 3.5 |
| 3a | **car** — water — **boat** | | 3c | car — **water** — **boat** | 6.0 |
| 3b | ***Why?*** transportation, take you places, go in them / drive them, have motors | 5.0 | 3d | ***Why?*** boat goes in / moves in / across water | 6.0 |
| 4a | **mother** — **father** — daughter | | 4c | **mother** — father — **daughter** | 5.0 |
| 4b | ***Why?*** married, parents, takes two to make a daughter | 4.5 | 4d | ***Why?*** females, girls, women, daughter comes from mother | 2.5 |

| Item | Item Content/Responses | Ability Score | Item | Item Content/Responses | Ability Score |
|---|---|---|---|---|---|
| 5a | **taste** — nose — **smell** | | 5c | taste — **nose** — **smell** | 6.0 |
| 5b | ***Why?*** both senses (**not**—you can smell and taste food) | 4.0 | 5d | ***Why?*** smell with nose, use nose to smell | 1.5 |

| Item | Item Content/Responses | Ability Score | Item | Item Content/Responses | Ability Score |
|---|---|---|---|---|---|
| 6a | painter — **elevator** — **ladder** | | 6c | **painter** — elevator — **ladder** | 5.0 |
| 6b | ***Why?*** use to go up and down / reach high places (**not**—go up only) | 5.0 | 6d | ***Why?*** painter uses / stands on ladder | 5.5 |

| Item | Item Content/Responses | Ability Score | Item | Item Content/Responses | Ability Score |
|---|---|---|---|---|---|
| 7a | bat — **eagle** — **owl** | | 7c | **bat** — eagle — **owl** | 6.0 |
| 7b | ***Why?*** both birds, have feathers | 7.5 | 7d | ***Why?*** nocturnal, up at night | 7.5 |

Time to administer: _____ **Subtotal Score 1** _____ / 34.5

**Subtotal Score 2** _____ / 66.0

**Subtotal Score 1** _____ / 34.5

**TOTAL WHAT GOES TOGETHER ABILTY SCORE** _____ / 100.5

**Behavioral observations:** (Abbreviations may be used next to items where they apply.)

___ Repetition of instructions (Rep)
___ Attention reminder required (Attn)
___ Prompt to reestablish set (Prompt)
___ Perseveration (P)
___ Delayed response (5+ sec) (DR)
___ Unintelligible response (UnR)
___ No response (NR)
___ I don't know (IDK)
___ Self-correction (SC)

**Additional qualitative/behavioral observations:**

**Notes for examiners on What Goes Together:** What Goes Together is a test of semantic/conceptual knowledge, categorical awareness, and mental flexibility. In addition to quantitative scoring of this task, you should write any nonallowed responses for qualitative information. Look for the following types of no-credit responses to "Why?": personalization (e.g., *"Because I have a mother and father"*), perseverative thought processes (e.g., *"A painter paints the ladder. A painter paints the elevator"*), emotional coloring (e.g., *"You kill with a knife and saw", "You kill an owl with a bat"*), generalizations (e.g., *"They're the same thing"*), and total failure to see a relationship (e.g., *"I don't know why"*).

## SUBTEST 5: DIGIT SPAN

**Materials** Test Form

**Instructions** Say, ***"I am going to say some numbers. Listen to the numbers, and when I finish, you say them back to me exactly the same way. Wait until I stop saying numbers before you begin."***

- Present numbers at the rate of 1 per second with even stress and prosody.
- Do not chunk numbers.
- No written responses are permitted on this subtest.

**Discontinue Rule** Discontinue if the child fails both sequences for any item and cross out scores for remaining items.

**Repetition** Not allowed

**Scoring**

- Cross out ability score for any incorrect item or for all items following discontinuation; circle ability score for each correct item.
- Add scores for correct items to compute total ability score.

| Item | Stimuli/Responses | Ability Score | Item | Stimuli/Responses | Ability Score |
|---|---|---|---|---|---|
| 1a | ***7 – 3*** | 0.5 | 1b | ***5 – 9*** | 0.5 |
| 2a | ***5 – 8 – 2*** | 0.5 | 2b | ***4 – 1 – 8*** | 1.0 |
| 3a | ***6 – 4 – 9 – 3*** | 4.0 | 3b | ***8 – 2 – 5 – 1*** | 5.0 |
| 4a | ***7 – 5 – 1 – 4 – 9*** | 9.5 | 4b | ***3 – 8 – 1 – 7 – 2*** | 10.0 |
| 5a | ***9 – 2 – 5 – 8 – 1 – 4*** | 11.5 | 5b | ***2 – 5 – 9 – 6 – 3 – 8*** | 12.5 |
| 6a | ***1 – 7 – 3 – 8 – 6 – 2 – 9*** | 13.5 | 6b | ***7 – 2 – 5 – 8 – 1 – 9 – 4*** | 14.0 |

Time to administer: _____ **Subtotal Score 1** _____ / 39.5

**Subtotal Score 2** _____ / 43.0

**Subtotal Score 1** _____ / 39.5

**TOTAL DIGIT SPAN ABILITY SCORE** _____ / 82.5

**Behavioral observations:** (Abbreviations may be used next to items where they apply.)

___ Repetition of instructions (Rep)
___ Attention reminder required (Attn)
___ Prompt to reestablish set (Prompt)
___ Perseveration (P)
___ Delayed response (5+ sec) (DR)
___ Unintelligible response (UnR)
___ No response (NR)
___ I don't know (IDK)
___ Self-correction (SC

**Additional qualitative/behavioral observations:**

**Notes for examiners on Digit Span:** Digit Span is primarily a test of attention and immediate memory. In the early phase of recovery, Digit Span performance may be below normal range but then recover independently of tasks with higher level cognitive demands. You can examine qualitative patterns by writing the numbers as spoken by examinees. Look for patterns such as repeating correct numbers in the wrong order, remembering only first numbers (primacy) or last numbers (recency) in longer strings, substituting overlearned sequences (e.g., 3, 4, 5), and perseverating on numbers from earlier responses. Remember that this task requires verbal production of exact words and examinees are not allowed to write responses; therefore, it may not be a valid task for individuals who cannot speak.

***NOTE: If you are administering this test in two sessions, end the first testing session here.***

**NOTE: *If you are administering this test in two sessions, start the second testing session here.***

## SUBTEST 6: NAMING

| | |
|---|---|
| **Materials** | Test Form, Stimulus Book (page 11) |
| **Instructions** | Open the Stimulus Book to page 11 and show the child the picture of the boy on his skateboard.<br>• Ask the child the question for each item in the table below while pointing to the precise location of the target item.<br>• If the child starts to elaborate, say, ***"Just give me one word."***<br>Record each response verbatim. If the child names an adjacent item, prompt, ***"No, this part."***<br>DO NOT tell the child to remember the picture for later. |
| **Discontinue Rule** | None |
| **Repetition** | Repeat the question one time if the child does not respond within 10 seconds. |
| **Scoring** | • Cross out ability score for any incorrect item; circle ability score for each correct item.<br>• Add scores for correct items to compute total ability score.<br>• Do not penalize dysarthria or recognizable mispronunciations (e.g., *eblow*). |

| Item | Question | Target Item/Response | Ability Score |
|---|---|---|---|
| 1 | ***What do you call these things?***<br>(If child names "trucks" [part of a skateboard], say, ***"No, this part,"*** and point again, specifically to wheels) | Wheels | 0.5 |
| 2 | ***What do you call these things?***<br>(If child names "laces" [or other part], say, ***"No, the whole thing."***) | Boots / Shoes | 0.5 |
| 3 | ***What do you call this thing?*** | Star | 0.5 |
| 4 | ***What do you call this thing?*** | Chain / ID tags / Dog tags / Necklace | 1.5 |
| 5 | ***What do you call this thing?*** | Band-Aid | 2.0 |
| 6 | ***What do you call this part of his body?*** | Chin | 2.0 |
| 7 | ***And this part of his body?*** | Elbow | 2.5 |
| 8 | ***And this part?***<br>(If child names "eye" [or other part], say, ***"No, this part."***) | Eyebrow | 3.0 |

Time to administer: _____ **TOTAL NAMING ABILITY SCORE** _____ / 12.5

**Behavioral observations:** (Abbreviations may be used next to items where they apply.)

| | | |
|---|---|---|
| ___ Repetition of instructions (Rep) | ___ Perseveration (P) | ___ No response (NR) |
| ___ Attention reminder required (Attn) | ___ Delayed response (5+ sec) (DR) | ___ I don't know (IDK) |
| ___ Prompt to reestablish set (Prompt) | ___ Unintelligible response (UnR) | ___ Self-correction (SC) |

**Additional qualitative/behavioral observations:**

**Notes for examiners on Naming:** Naming deficits are a key symptom of aphasia, and even delayed retrieval may be a sign of mild anomia. By recording an examinee's exact responses, you can identify error types such as semantic paraphasias (e.g., "ankle" for *elbow*), phonemic paraphasias (e.g., "eyetrow" for *eyebrow*), and circumlocutions (e.g., "put it around your neck" for *necklace/chain*), as well as perseverations. Look also for verbosity (elaboration rather than naming the item). In such cases, say, ***"Just give me one word."*** When misnaming occurs, try to identify the mechanism(s) for the error (e.g., language problem, visual acuity, visual perceptual deficits). In addition to testing naming ability, this subtest has a secondary purpose, which is to draw the examinee's attention to key elements of the picture for later recall (Subtest 9: Picture Recall). If the child comments on the danger of the skateboarder wearing a hat rather than a helmet, say, ***"You're absolutely right."***

## SUBTEST 7: STORY RETELLING—IMMEDIATE

**Materials**

Test Form, for children in:

**Grades 1–3:** Read Story 1, "Bobby's Lucky Day."
**Grades 4–7:** Read Story 2, "Tommy the Trickster."
**Grades 8–11:** Read Story 3, "The Rock Concert."

**Instructions**

Say, ***"I'm going to tell you a story. Listen carefully. I want you to repeat the whole story back to me exactly as I told it to you. I can only read it once. Are you ready?"*** Although "exactly" is in the instructions to the child, some semantically acceptable substitutions, as indicated, can receive credit.

***"Okay, here is the story."*** Use natural inflection when reading the story.

After reading the story, say, ***"Now tell me the same story. Start now."***

*Probe:* If the child does not initiate the story, say, ***"What was the story about? What happened?"***

DO NOT tell the child to remember the story for later.

**Discontinue Rule**

None

**Repetition**

Repeat the directions one time if requested.

Prompt as indicated if the child does not begin retelling the story within 10 seconds.

**Scoring**

- Identify each correct story element recalled and circle corresponding ability score; cross out ability score for any omitted or incorrect item.
- Count acceptable semantic substitutions as correct.
- Do not count variations that change the meaning (e.g., "street" for *sidewalk*).
- Count pronouns as correct; but at first mention, the child must say characters' proper names (*Bobby, Tommy, Daryl, Rochelle*).
- Count elements told out of sequence as correct.
- Add scores for correct items to compute total ability score.

### STORY 1 (GRADES 1–3)

Read the following story: "Bobby's Lucky Day"

***"Bobby's grandmother gave him some money to buy candy. On his way to the store, the money fell out of a hole in his pocket. Bobby was really upset. But suddenly, he saw a dollar on the sidewalk in front of the store. It was Bobby's lucky day!"***

Say, ***"Now tell me the same story. Start now."***

*Probe:* If the child does not initiate the story, say, ***"What was the story about? What happened?"***

| Item | **Story Elements** (optional wording) | Ability Score | Item | **Story Elements** (optional wording) | Ability Score |
|---|---|---|---|---|---|
| 1 | Bobby's (must use proper name to count) | 0.5 | 12 | in his pocket | 1.0 |
| 2 | grandmother | 2.0 | 13 | Bobby (he) | 3.0 |
| 3 | gave him (Bobby) | 1.5 | 14 | (really) upset / mad | 4.0 |
| 4 | (some) money | 1.0 | 15 | but suddenly | 5.5 |
| 5 | to buy | 3.0 | 16 | he (Bobby) saw | 1.5 |
| 6 | candy | 3.0 | 17 | a dollar | 1.0 |
| 7 | on his way to | 4.0 | 18 | on the sidewalk | 3.0 |
| 8 | the store | 3.0 | 19 | in front of | 3.0 |
| 9 | (the) money | 2.5 | 20 | the store | 2.5 |
| 10 | fell out of | 1.5 | 21 | Bobby's (his) | 1.5 |
| 11 | a hole | 2.0 | 22 | lucky day | 1.5 |

Time to administer: _____ **Subtotal Score 1** _____ / 24.0

**Subtotal Score 2** _____ / 27.5

**Subtotal Score 1** _____ / 24.0

**TOTAL STORY RETELLING—IMMEDIATE ABILTY SCORE** _____ / 51.5

## STORY 2 (GRADES 4–7)

Read the following story: "Tommy the Trickster"

***"Tommy's mother thought he was getting fat from eating too much junk food, so she stocked the refrigerator with fruit and carrot sticks. She even put these things in his lunchbox. But Tommy was a fast talker. At school he convinced his friends that cookies were bad for them. Then he traded his fruit and carrots for their cookies. His mother didn't know why Tommy kept gaining weight when all she had given him were healthy foods."***

Say, ***"Now tell me the same story. Start now."***

*Probe:* If the child does not initiate the story, say, ***"What was the story about? What happened?"***

| Item | Story Elements (optional wording) | Ability Score |
|---|---|---|
| 1 | Tommy's (must use proper name to count) | 0.5 |
| 2 | mother | 2.0 |
| 3 | thought he (Tommy) | 4.0 |
| 4 | was getting fat (bigger, gaining weight) | 1.0 |
| 5 | from eating | 5.5 |
| 6 | too much | 6.0 |
| 7 | junk food | 5.5 |
| 8 | so she | 4.0 |
| 9 | stocked | 5.0 |
| 10 | the refrigerator | 4.5 |
| 11 | fruit (healthy foods) (only scores once) | 4.5 |
| 12 | carrot (sticks) (healthy foods) | 5.0 |
| 13 | she even put | 5.5 |
| 14 | these things | 6.0 |
| 15 | in his lunch box | 5.0 |
| 16 | but Tommy (he) | 4.5 |
| 17 | was a "fast talker" (figurative meaning) | 6.0 |

Time to administer: _____ **Subtotal Score 1** _____ / 74.5

| Item | Story Elements (optional wording) | Ability Score |
|---|---|---|
| 18 | at school | 5.5 |
| 19 | he convinced (talked them into, told) | 4.0 |
| 20 | his friends | 3.5 |
| 21 | that cookies | 2.0 |
| 22 | were bad | 3.5 |
| 23 | for them | 3.5 |
| 24 | then he traded | 2.0 |
| 25 | his fruit | 5.5 |
| 26 | carrots | 6.0 |
| 27 | cookies | 4.5 |
| 28 | his mother | 3.5 |
| 29 | didn't know why | 4.0 |
| 30 | Tommy (he) | 4.5 |
| 31 | kept gaining weight (getting bigger / fatter) | 4.0 |
| 32 | when all she had given him | 6.0 |
| 33 | were healthy foods | 6.0 |

**Subtotal Score 2** _____ / 68.0

**Subtotal Score 1** _____ / 74.5

**TOTAL STORY RETELLING—IMMEDIATE ABILTY SCORE** _____ / 142.5

**Notes for examiners on Story Retelling—Immediate:** Story Retelling—Immediate calls upon various cognitive and linguistic skills, most importantly, memory and higher level discourse ability. Three levels of PTBI™ stories are provided to hold interest for individuals at different grade levels. You should check off and score stated story elements and also transcribe the language sample for purposes of qualitative review. Look for perseverative thought processes, misnaming of characters, personalization, elaboration and confabulation, primacy effects (better recall of the first part of story), and recency effects (better recall of end of story). Compare performance on this task with that on Story Retelling—Delayed to note ability to consolidate, remember, and retrieve recently heard information.

## STORY 3 (GRADES 8–11)

Read the following story: "The Rock Concert"

***"Last spring, Daryl got two free tickets to an outdoor rock concert. So, he asked his friend Rochelle to go with him. Daryl said to his father, 'If you let me go to the concert with Rochelle and drive us there, I will take out the trash for three months.' Rochelle said to her mother, 'If you let me go to the concert with Daryl and pick us up afterwards, I promise to babysit my sister six times.' Both parents agreed. Ten minutes after the kids were dropped off, it began to pour. The concert was cancelled. The kids couldn't believe it. They would still have to keep their promises!"***

Say, ***"Now tell me the same story. Start now."***

*Probe:* If the child does not initiate the story, say, ***"What was the story about? What happened?"***

| Item | Story Elements (optional wording) | Ability Score | Item | Story Elements (optional wording) | Ability Score |
|---|---|---|---|---|---|
| 1 | Last spring | 4.5 | 23 | months | 2.5 |
| 2 | Daryl got (must use proper name to count) | 2.0 | 24 | Rochelle (she) said | 4.0 |
| 3 | two | 3.0 | 25 | to her mother | 4.0 |
| 4 | free | 4.0 | 26 | if you let me go (allow me to go) | 3.5 |
| 5 | tickets to | 1.5 | 27 | and pick us up afterwards | 1.0 |
| 6 | outdoor | 5.0 | 28 | I promise | 2.5 |
| 7 | rock | 2.5 | 29 | to babysit | 2.5 |
| 8 | concert | 0.5 | 30 | my sister | 5.0 |
| 9 | so he asked | 2.5 | 31 | six times | 5.0 |
| 10 | his friend | 3.0 | 32 | both parents | 5.0 |
| 11 | Rochelle (must use proper name to count) | 3.0 | 33 | agreed | 5.0 |
| 12 | to go | 3.5 | 34 | ten | 4.0 |
| 13 | with him | 4.0 | 35 | minutes | 3.5 |
| 14 | Daryl (he) said | 3.0 | 36 | after the kids | 1.0 |
| 15 | to his father | 2.0 | 37 | were dropped off | 2.5 |
| 16 | if you let me go | 3.0 | 38 | it began to "pour" (rain) | 2.0 |
| 17 | to the concert | 3.5 | 39 | the concert | 3.0 |
| 18 | with Rochelle (her) | 3.5 | 40 | was cancelled | 5.5 |
| 19 | and drive us (there) (give us a ride) | 4.0 | 41 | the kids (they) | 2.0 |
| 20 | I will take out | 2.0 | 42 | couldn't believe it (**not**—they were mad) | 5.5 |
| 21 | the trash (garbage) | 3.0 | 43 | would still have to | 2.0 |
| 22 | three | 2.5 | 44 | keep their promises (do their jobs) | 2.0 |

Time to administer: _____ **Subtotal Score 1** _____ / 65.5

**Subtotal Score 2** _____ / 73.0

**Subtotal Score 1** _____ / 65.5

**TOTAL STORY RETELLING—IMMEDIATE ABILTY SCORE** _____ / 138.5

**Behavioral observations:** (Abbreviations may be used next to items where they apply.)

___ Repetition of instructions (Rep)
___ Attention reminder required (Attn)
___ Prompt to reestablish set (Prompt)
___ Perseveration (P)
___ Delayed response (5+ sec) (DR)
___ Unintelligible response (UnR)
___ No response (NR)
___ I don't know (IDK)
___ Self-correction (SC)

**Additional qualitative/behavioral observations:**

## SUBTEST 8: YES/NO/MAYBE

**Materials** Test Form, Stimulus Book (pages 12–17)

**Instructions** Open the Stimulus Book to page 12 in front of the child.

Say, ***"Now we're going to read some very short stories together. I'll read and you follow along."*** (If the child can read aloud and wants to, let him or her do so. Do not require choral reading.)

Say, ***"Pay careful attention, because I'm going to ask you some questions after each story. Your answer can be 'yes' if you are certain the answer is 'yes,' or 'no' if you are certain the answer is 'no.' If the story doesn't clearly tell you the answer, you should say 'maybe.' Here is a practice item."***

- Do not remove the Stimulus Book; keep it in front of the child.
- Circle *Y* for "yes," *N* for "no," and *M* for "maybe" answers. Correct answers are in bold on the Test Form.

*Note:* If the child is unable to speak, write YES NO MAYBE in a vertical array on a piece of paper to allow a pointing response.

**Discontinue Rule** Discontinue testing if the child cannot get into set for the task after coaching on the practice story or if the child misses all items on two consecutive stories.

**Repetition** Only allowed during the practice story

**Scoring**

- Score self-corrections as correct only if immediate.
- Circle ability score for correct items; cross out ability score for incorrect items or items following discontinuation.
- Add subtotals for each short story.
- Compute total ability score by adding the story subscores.

**Practice Story** Say, ***"One morning, Susan missed the school bus. She thought she would be late for school, but her mother got her there on time."*** Say, ***"I can help you read it again if you want."***

Reread the practice story as often as requested, and then ask the following questions. Reinforce the correct answer for each practice question, and help the child to see the relationship if necessary.

| | | | | |
|---|---|---|---|---|
| a | ***"Did Susan miss the bus?"*** | **(Y)** | N | M |
| b | ***"Was Susan late for school?"*** | Y | **(N)** | M |
| c | ***"Was it raining that morning?"*** | Y | N | **(M)** |
| d | ***"Did her father take her to school?"*** | Y | **(N)** | M |

**Short Story 1** (Turn to page 13 in the Stimulus Book. *Note:* This story has only three questions.)

***The kids ran after the blue ice cream truck. It turned the corner before they could catch it.***

| Item | Questions | Responses | Ability Score |
|---|---|---|---|
| a | ***Did the kids chase the ice cream truck?*** | **(Y)** N M | 0.5 |
| b | ***Did the kids catch the truck before it turned the corner?*** | Y **(N)** M | 0.5 |
| c | ***Was the ice cream truck red?*** | Y **(N)** M | 0.5 |

**Story 1 Ability Score** _____ / 1.5

**Short Story 2** (Turn to page 14 in the Stimulus Book.)

***"What I did on my summer vacation" is the topic the teacher makes her class write about on the first day of school every year. When school started a month ago, the teacher gave her usual first writing assignment.***

| Item | Questions | Responses | Ability Score |
|---|---|---|---|
| a | ***Did the teacher ask her class to write about their summer vacations?*** | **(Y)** N M | 0.5 |
| b | ***Was the Middle East the first writing topic of the year?*** | Y **(N)** M | 3.5 |
| c | ***Did school start last week?*** | Y **(N)** M | 1.0 |
| d | ***Did all of the students take a trip on their summer vacations?*** | Y N **(M)** | 2.0 |

**Story 2 Ability Score** _____ / 7.0
**Story 1 Ability Score** _____ / 1.5
**Subtotal Score** _____ / 8.5

| **Short Story 3** (Turn to page 15 in the Stimulus Book.) | | | |
|---|---|---|---|
| ***Immanuel was the first one of a small group of boys in his class who could dunk a basketball.*** | | | |
| **Item** | **Questions** | **Responses** | **Ability Score** |
| a | ***Could Immanuel jump the highest in class?*** | Y N **(M)** | 1.0 |
| b | ***Could some of the other boys dunk a basketball?*** | **(Y)** N M | 2.5 |
| c | ***Could all of the boys in Immanuel's class dunk a basketball?*** | Y **(N)** M | 2.5 |
| d | ***Was Immanuel the best basketball player in his class?*** | Y N **(M)** | 2.0 |

**Story 3 Ability Score** _____ / 8.0

| **Short Story 4** (Turn to page 16 in the Stimulus Book.) | | | |
|---|---|---|---|
| ***Mary and Todd decided they would go to the beach on Saturday even if it was a cloudy day. When they woke up on Saturday, it was sunny.*** | | | |
| **Item** | **Questions** | **Responses** | **Ability Score** |
| a | ***Did Mary and Todd plan to go to the beach on Saturday if it was cloudy?*** | **(Y)** N M | 2.0 |
| b | ***Did it rain later on Saturday?*** | Y N **(M)** | 4.0 |
| c | ***Was it cloudy when Mary and Todd woke up on Saturday?*** | Y **(N)** M | 2.5 |
| d | ***Was Mary the mother of Todd?*** | Y N **(M)** | 2.0 |

**Story 4 Ability Score** _____ / 10.5

| **Short Story 5** (Turn to page 17 in the Stimulus Book.) | | | |
|---|---|---|---|
| ***The scientists observed the insects closely over a 24-hour period, hoping to study their swarming behavior. At that point, the scientists concluded that the insects had been prevented from swarming because of the unusual atmospheric conditions.*** | | | |
| **Item** | **Questions** | **Responses** | **Ability Score** |
| a | ***Did the insects swarm?*** | Y **(N)** M | 4.5 |
| b | ***Did the scientists watch the insects for a full day?*** | **(Y)** N M | 0.5 |
| c | ***Can atmospheric conditions influence the swarming of insects?*** | **(Y)** N M | 2.5 |
| d | ***Did the scientists accomplish their original goal?*** | Y **(N)** M | 4.5 |

Time to administer _____

**Story 5 Ability Score** _____ / 12.0
**Story 4 Ability Score** _____ / 10.5
**Story 3 Ability Score** _____ / 8.0
**Subtotal from page 14** _____ / 8.5
**TOTAL YES/NO/MAYBE ABILITY SCORE** _____ / 39.0

**Behavioral observations:** (Abbreviations may be used next to items where they apply.)

| | | |
|---|---|---|
| ___ Repetition of instructions (Rep) | ___ Perseveration (P) | ___ No response (NR) |
| ___ Attention reminder required (Attn) | ___ Delayed response (5+ sec) (DR) | ___ I don't know (IDK) |
| ___ Prompt to reestablish set (Prompt) | ___ Unintelligible response (UnR) | ___ Self-correction (SC) |

**Additional qualitative/behavioral observations:**

**Notes for examiners on Yes/No/Maybe:** The Yes/No/Maybe subtest was designed to test the ability to listen to/read short stories carefully enough to answer questions regarding both stated and inferred information. As such, this subtest requires several cognitive processes, including higher level language comprehension skills, attention, and mental tracking. In addition to computing the overall ability score, look for error patterns such as missing "maybe" responses or perseverating on one answer choice.

## SUBTEST 9: PICTURE RECALL

**Materials** Test Form, Stimulus Book (page 11)

**Instructions** Say, ***"Remember the picture of the boy that I showed you a while ago?"*** If the child can't recall the picture, cue by saying, ***"The one where you named some parts of his body and other things."*** Then say, ***"Please draw that boy on this page."***

Use the last page of this Test Form.

Say, ***"Put in as many details as you can remember."***

*Probe:* If the child still can't remember the picture, say to the child, ***"Just draw a picture of any boy."***

When the child is finished or you see that he or she is not being productive, say, ***"Now we need your autograph. Please sign your first and last name on the bottom of your picture. Write it clearly so that anyone could read it."*** (Point to the bottom of the page.)

*Probe:* Okay to probe for last name if only first name is given.

*Probe:* If the picture is unclear or if the child is unable to draw, ask for a description, write down what the child says, and score recalled elements.

If the child cannot move to write his or her name, ask for a spelling. All letters in the name must be correct to receive credit.

**Discontinue Rule** If the child does not respond after 10 seconds following allowed prompting, discontinue.

**Repetition** If the child does not respond within 10 seconds, repeat the instructions and use the probe.

**Scoring**

- Circle ability score for any component recognizable in context.
- Cross out ability score for any missing component.
- All letters in name must be legible and correct for name to receive credit.
- Add subtotals for each column.
- Compute total ability score by adding the column subtotals.

| Item | Picture Recall | Ability Score |
|---|---|---|
| 1 | Picture of a boy | 1.5 |
| 2 | Skateboard | 3.0 |
| 3 | Hat / Baseball cap | 5.5 |
| 4 | Boots / Shoes | 5.5 |
| 5 | Star | 6.0 |
| 6 | Chain / ID tags / Dog tags / Necklace | 6.0 |
| 7 | Band-Aid | 7.0 |
| 8 | Shorts | 7.5 |

**Picture Recall Subtotal** _____ / 42.0

| Item | Signature | Ability Score |
|---|---|---|
| 1 | First name | 0.5 |
| 2 | Last name | 3.0 |

**Signature Subtotal** _____ / 3.5

**Picture Recall Subtotal** _____ / 42.0

**TOTAL PICTURE RECALL ABILITY SCORE** _____ / 45.5

Time to administer: _____

Hand used: _____ L _____ R

**Behavioral observations:** (Abbreviations may be used next to items where they apply.)

| | | |
|---|---|---|
| ___ Repetition of instructions (Rep) | ___ Perseveration (P) | ___ No response (NR) |
| ___ Attention reminder required (Attn) | ___ Delayed response (5+ sec) (DR) | ___ I don't know (IDK) |
| ___ Prompt to reestablish set (Prompt) | ___ Unintelligible response (UnR) | ___ Self-correction (SC |

**Additional qualitative/behavioral observations:**

**Notes for examiners on Picture Recall:** This subtest assesses incidental memory (i.e., without instruction to remember) for the picture presented in Subtest 6 and ability to depict recalled elements of that picture (through drawing, or speaking, in the case of individuals who are unable to hold a pen). The recalled components are scored, but it is important that you study the picture carefully and look for such features as micrographia (tiny drawing), proportionality, perseverative elements, unilateral neglect (drawing only half the picture), and fragmentation (refer to the *PTBI™ Examiner's Manual* for examples). Signatures as well as spelling can be analyzed for some of these same features.

## SUBTEST 10: STORY RETELLING—DELAYED

**Materials** Test Form, for children in:
**Grades 1–3:** Score Story 1, "Bobby's Lucky Day."
**Grades 4–7:** Score Story 2, "Tommy the Trickster."
**Grades 8–11:** Score Story 3, "The Rock Concert."

**Instructions** Do not reread the story. The child must recall the story from the prior experience.

Say, ***"Remember the story [title of story child heard]? Tell me the story again. Try to remember as much as you can."***

As the child retells the story, check story elements recalled correctly or record verbatim any content variations in the story produced.

**Discontinue Rule** None

**Repetition** Repeat the directions one time if requested.

**Scoring**
- Identify each correct story element recalled and circle corresponding ability score; cross out ability score for any omitted or incorrect item.
- Count acceptable semantic substitutions as correct.
- Do not count variations that change the meaning (e.g., "street" for *sidewalk*).
- Count pronouns as correct; but at first mention, the child must say characters' proper names (*Bobby, Tommy, Daryl, Rochelle).*
- Count elements told out of sequence as correct.
- Add scores for correct items to compute total ability score.

### STORY 1 (GRADES 1–3)

Say, ***"Remember the story 'Bobby's Lucky Day'? Tell me the story again. Try to remember as much as you can"***

| Item | **Story Elements** (optional wording) | Ability Score |
|---|---|---|
| 1 | Bobby's (must use proper name to count) | 1.5 |
| 2 | grandmother | 1.5 |
| 3 | gave him (Bobby) | 1.5 |
| 4 | (some) money | 1.5 |
| 5 | to buy | 3.5 |
| 6 | candy | 3.5 |
| 7 | on his way to | 4.0 |
| 8 | the store | 3.0 |
| 9 | (the) money | 2.0 |
| 10 | fell out of | 1.5 |
| 11 | a hole | 2.0 |

Time to administer: _____ **Subtotal Score 1** _____ / 25.5

| Item | **Story Elements** (optional wording) | Ability Score |
|---|---|---|
| 12 | in his pocket | 1.0 |
| 13 | Bobby (he) | 3.5 |
| 14 | (really) upset / mad | 4.5 |
| 15 | but suddenly | 5.5 |
| 16 | he (Bobby) saw | 0.5 |
| 17 | a dollar | 0.5 |
| 18 | on the sidewalk | 3.0 |
| 19 | in front of | 3.5 |
| 20 | the store | 2.5 |
| 21 | Bobby's (his) | 2.0 |
| 22 | lucky day | 2.0 |

**Subtotal Score 2** _____ / 28.5

**Subtotal Score 1** _____ / 25.5

**TOTAL STORY RETELLING—DELAYED ABILTY SCORE** _____ / 54.0

## STORY 2 (GRADES 4–7)

Say, ***"Remember the story 'Tommy the Trickster'? Tell me the story again. Try to remember as much as you can."***

| Item | **Story Elements** (optional wording) | Ability Score |
|---|---|---|
| 1 | Tommy's (must use proper name to count) | 1.0 |
| 2 | mother | 1.0 |
| 3 | thought he (Tommy) | 2.0 |
| 4 | was getting fat (bigger, gaining weight) | 0.5 |
| 5 | from eating | 3.5 |
| 6 | too much | 5.0 |
| 7 | junk food | 4.0 |
| 8 | so she | 2.0 |
| 9 | stocked | 2.5 |
| 10 | the refrigerator | 2.0 |
| 11 | fruit (healthy foods) [only scores once] | 2.5 |
| 12 | carrot (sticks) (healthy foods) | 2.5 |
| 13 | she even put | 3.5 |
| 14 | these things | 4.0 |
| 15 | in his lunch box | 3.0 |
| 16 | but Tommy (he) | 3.0 |
| 17 | was a "fast talker" (figurative meaning) | 4.0 |

Time to administer: _____ **Subtotal Score 1** _____ / 46.0

| Item | **Story Elements** (optional wording) | Ability Score |
|---|---|---|
| 18 | at school | 3.0 |
| 19 | he convinced (talked them into, told) | 2.0 |
| 20 | his friends | 1.5 |
| 21 | that cookies | 1.0 |
| 22 | were bad | 1.5 |
| 23 | for them | 2.5 |
| 24 | then he traded | 1.5 |
| 25 | his fruit | 3.5 |
| 26 | carrots | 3.5 |
| 27 | cookies | 2.5 |
| 28 | his mother | 1.0 |
| 29 | didn't know why | 2.0 |
| 30 | Tommy (he) | 2.0 |
| 31 | kept gaining weight (getting bigger / fatter) | 1.5 |
| 32 | when all she had given him | 4.0 |
| 33 | were healthy foods | 4.0 |

**Subtotal Score 2** _____ / 37.0

**Subtotal Score 1** _____ / 46.0

**TOTAL STORY RETELLING—DELAYED ABILTY SCORE** _____ / 83.0

**Notes for examiners on Story Retelling—Delayed:** As indicated in the note to examiners for Subtest 7 (Story Retelling—Immediate), complex narrative skills are needed for story retelling. Possible recall patterns and error types are also described there. It is important to compare performance on the immediate and delayed recall tasks to observe ability to consolidate, remember, and retrieve information that was just heard versus information heard some time before. Like Subtest 9 (Picture Recall), this is a test of incidental memory, as examinees are not told to remember the story the first time they hear it.

## STORY 3 (GRADES 8–11)

Say, ***"Remember the story 'The Rock Concert'? Tell me the story again. Try to remember as much as you can."***

| Item | **Story Elements** (optional wording) | Ability Score |
|---|---|---|
| 1 | Last spring | 4.0 |
| 2 | Daryl got (must use proper name to count) | 2.0 |
| 3 | two | 2.5 |
| 4 | free | 4.0 |
| 5 | tickets to | 1.0 |
| 6 | outdoor | 4.5 |
| 7 | rock | 1.5 |
| 8 | concert | 0.5 |
| 9 | so he asked | 2.0 |
| 10 | his friend | 2.5 |
| 11 | Rochelle (must use proper name to count) | 2.5 |
| 12 | to go | 2.5 |
| 13 | with him | 3.5 |
| 14 | Daryl (he) said | 2.5 |
| 15 | to his father | 1.5 |
| 16 | if you let me go | 3.0 |
| 17 | to the concert | 4.0 |
| 18 | with Rochelle (her) | 4.5 |
| 19 | and drive us (there) (give us a ride) | 3.0 |
| 20 | I will take out | 1.5 |
| 21 | the trash (garbage) | 1.0 |
| 22 | three | 2.5 |

Time to administer: _____ **Subtotal Score 1** _____ / 56.5

| Item | **Story Elements** (optional wording) | Ability Score |
|---|---|---|
| 23 | months | 2.5 |
| 24 | Rochelle (she) said | 2.5 |
| 25 | to her mother | 1.5 |
| 26 | if you let me go (allow me to go) | 3.0 |
| 27 | and pick us up afterwards | 3.0 |
| 28 | I promise | 2.5 |
| 29 | to babysit | 1.0 |
| 30 | my sister | 2.5 |
| 31 | six times | 2.5 |
| 32 | both parents | 4.0 |
| 33 | agreed | 3.5 |
| 34 | ten | 3.5 |
| 35 | minutes | 3.5 |
| 36 | after the kids | 3.0 |
| 37 | were dropped off | 3.0 |
| 38 | it began to "pour" (rain) | 1.0 |
| 39 | the concert | 1.0 |
| 40 | was cancelled | 1.5 |
| 41 | the kids (they) | 3.0 |
| 42 | couldn't believe it (**not**—they were mad) | 3.5 |
| 43 | would still have to | 1.5 |
| 44 | keep their promises (do their jobs) | 1.5 |

**Subtotal Score 2** _____ / 54.5

**Subtotal Score 1** _____ / 56.5

**TOTAL STORY RETELLING—DELAYED ABILTY SCORE** _____ / 111.0

**Behavioral observations:** (Abbreviations may be used next to items where they apply.)

___ Repetition of instructions (Rep)
___ Attention reminder required (Attn)
___ Prompt to reestablish set (Prompt)
___ Perseveration (P)
___ Delayed response (5+ sec) (DR)
___ Unintelligible response (UnR)
___ No response (NR)
___ I don't know (IDK)
___ Self-correction (SC)

**Additional qualitative/behavioral observations:**

· P A U L · H ·
BROOKES
PUBLISHING CO.®
www.brookespublishing.com

This Test Form is sold as one in a package under
ISBN-13: 978-1-59857-109-7 / ISBN-10: 1-59857-109-5.

# SUBTEST 9: PICTURE RECALL

·P A U L·H·
BROOKES
PUBLISHING Co®
www.brookespublishing.com

This Test Form is sold as one in a package under
ISBN-13: 978-1-59857-109-7 / ISBN-10: 1-59857-109-5.

